ESSENTIAL GUIDE TO PSORIASIS

Understanding, Managing, and Thriving: An In-Depth Exploration of Psoriasis

DR. CASEY LOREN

© 2024 by CASEY LOREN

All rights reserved .Except for brief quotations included in critical reviews and certain other noncommercial uses allowed by copyright law, no part of this book may be reproduced, distributed, or transmitted in any form or by any means, including photocopying, recording, or other electronic or mechanical methods, without the publisher's prior written permission.

DISCLAIMER

This book's content is only meant to be used for general informative purposes. Although the author has taken great care to ensure the content is accurate and thorough, no warranties or assurances on the information's accuracy, correctness, or reliability are provided. It is recommended that readers employ their own judgment and discretion when applying any material found in this book to their particular situation.

The information in this book is not intended to replace professional advice, nor is the author an expert in any of the subjects covered. It is recommended that readers consult with experienced professionals regarding any particular issues or concerns.

Any name that may be mentioned or referred in this book does not imply endorsement, recommendation, or relationship on the part of the author with any person, entity, good, website, or association. These references are made only for informational purposes and are not meant to be taken as recommendations or endorsements.

The information contained in this book may cause readers to suffer loss or damage, for which the author disclaims all obligation and accountability. The only people accountable for the decisions and actions taken by readers using the information presented are themselves.

Any names, characters, companies, locations, activities, occasions, and incidents referenced in this book are either made up or the result of the author's imagination. Any likeness to real people, living or dead, or to real things is entirely coincidental.

This book's content may change at any time, without prior notice, according to the author. The onus is on the reader to verify whether there have been any updates or revisions.

The reader accepts the conditions of this disclaimer by reading this book. Please do not read this book or use its contents if you do not agree to these terms.

Table of Contents

CHAPTER 1 14

   GETTING TO KNOW PSORIASIS 14

   What is Psoriasis and What Are Its Symptoms 14

   What Causes It All 14

   The Signs and Prognosis 15

   Mental Health **Impact** 15

   Typical Errors 16

   Children Affected with Psoriasis 16

   Arthritis Psoriatic 17

   Causes of Danger 17

   News in the Field and Current Therapies 17

   Managing One's Lifestyle 18

CHAPTER 2 20

   PSORIASIS: A SCIENTIFIC PERSPECTIVE 20

   Psoriasis and the Immune System: 20

   The Role of Heredity: 20

Illness and Its Function: 21

The Life Cycle of Skin Cells: 21

Immune Factor: 22

Factors Influencing the Environment: 22

Conditions that occur together: 23

Social and psychological aspects: 23

The Role of Hormones: 24

New Treatment Options: 24

CHAPTER 3 26

HANDLING INTENSE PSORIASIS EPISODES 26

The Definitive Resource for Psoriasis: Flare-Up Management 26

Things to Steer Clear of 26

Nutrition and Diet Advice 29

Daily Skincare Programme 31

Sun Protection Recommendations 32

Physical fitness and regular exercise 32

Non-Conventional Medical Help 35

Resilience Techniques 36

CHAPTER 4 40
PSORIASIS MEDICAL TREATMENTS 40

Psoriasis Essentials: A Medical Professional's Guide to Treatments 40

Aesthetic Remedies 40

Photographic therapy 42

Medications in the System 43

Biologic medications 44

Treatments in Combination 45

Drugs administered intravenously 45

Medications Taken Orally 46

Guidelines for Treatment 47

CHAPTER 5 50
COMPREHENSIVE METHODS FOR TREATING PSORIASIS 50

Meditation and Mindfulness 50

Acupressure and Acupuncture 52

Natural Treatments 53

Numerous Ayurvedic Methods 54

fragrance treatment 55

Treatments using Homoeopathy 57

Doing Tai Chi and Yoga 58

Massage Treatments 59

Natural Health Care 60

Integrative health care 61

CHAPTER 6 64

EMOTIONAL WELL-BEING AND PSORIASIS 64

Psoriasis's Effect on Mental Health 64

Dealing with Difficult Emotions 64

Counselling and Support Groups 65

Methods for Reducing Stress 65

Developing Confidence 65

De-escalating Depression and Anxiety 66

Mental-Physical Link 66

Activities for Healing 67

Considering Expert Advice 67

CHAPTER 7 70

UNIQUE GROUPS AFFECTED BY PSORIASIS 70

Exploring Psoriasis During Pregnancy 70

Treatment for Psoriasis in Children 71

Psoriasis in the Elderly 71

Disparities between the Sexes and Psoriasis 72

Psoriasis Among Diverse Ethnic Communities 73

Psoriasis and the LGBTQ+ Community 73

Treatment of Psoriasis in Long-Term Conditions 74

Psoriasis and Being Overweight 75

Psoriasis's Effects on Sexual Health 75

Things to Think About at Work 76

CHAPTER 8 78

WAYS TO MANAGE PSORIASIS IN YOUR DAILY LIFE 78

The Definitive Resource for Living Well with Psoriasis 78

Quitting Smoking and Alcohol 78

Tips for Taking Care of Your Skin 79

Options for Attire..79

Changes to the Environment 80

Overcoming Psoriasis on the Road 80

Caring for Your Money...........................80

Emotional Well-being and Eczema 81

Relationship Management.....................81

Thoughts on What May Come Next 82

CHAPTER 9..84

HEALTHCARE SYSTEM NAVIGATION.....84

Choosing a Reliable Medical Professional ...84

Successfully Interacting with Medical Professionals..84

Expert Opinions and Second Opinions........85

Insurance Coverage Made Clear................... 85

Getting Drugs and Treatments..................... 86

Patient Rights and Advocacy....................... 86

Online Medical Care and Health Technology
.... 87

Clinical Trials and Involvement in Research
.... 88

Medical Facilities and Urgent Care............... 88

Planning for the End of Life 89

CHAPTER 10 90

TAKING CONTROL OF YOUR PSORIASIS 90

Resources for Learning and Research .. 90

Taking Responsibility for Your Health 90

Setting Achievable Objectives 91

Developing a System of Mutual Assistance .. 91

Raising Awareness about Psoriasis 92

The Importance of Prioritising Your Health 92

"Rejoicing in Success"................................. 93

Sustaining Oneself and Being Flexible.........93

Discovering Happiness and Success.....93

Managing Psoriasis in a Healthy Way...94

CHAPTER 1

GETTING TO KNOW PSORIASIS

What is Psoriasis and What Are Its Symptoms

A persistent autoimmune skin illness known as psoriasis causes the skin to produce more skin cells than it needs, resulting in thick, red, and scaly areas. Psoriasis comes in various forms, the most prevalent of which is plaque psoriasis. Other varieties include guttate, inverted, pustular, and erythrodermic psoriasis. Depending on the type, a patient may need a customized treatment plan.

What Causes It All

While researchers still don't know for sure what triggers psoriasis, they think it has something to do with the immune system, the environment, and genes. Stress, infections, skin injuries, certain drugs (such as lithium and beta-blockers), and changes in environment or weather can all worsen the symptoms of psoriasis.

The Signs and Prognosis

Red patches of skin covered in silvery scales; dry, cracked skin that bleeds; itching, burning, or pain; swollen or ridged nails; these are some of the symptoms of psoriasis, though they can vary in type and intensity. In most cases, a doctor will look at the patient's medical history, conduct a skin biopsy, and then diagnose based on that.

Mental Health **Impact**

Mental health can be greatly affected by living with psoriasis. Because the illness is apparent, people may experience emotions of shame, low self-esteem, and self-consciousness. A lot of people who have psoriasis also deal with sadness, anxiety, and feeling alone. One way to cope with the psychological effects of psoriasis is to reach out for help from people you care about, including healthcare providers, support groups, and loved ones.

Typical Errors

Among the many myths surrounding psoriasis are the following: that it is contagious; that it mostly affects the skin; that it can also impact the nails, joints, and other organs; and that it is purely a cosmetic concern; in reality, it is a chronic medical disorder that can have systemic implications. The best way to combat the stigmatization of psoriasis and refute these myths is by increasing public understanding and education.

Children Affected with Psoriasis

Children can also be affected by psoriasis, although it is more typically diagnosed in adults. Psoriasis in children may manifest differently from that in adults and may necessitate a different approach to treatment. To properly manage the illness in children, parents and carers must collaborate closely with healthcare specialists.

Arthritis Psoriatic

People who suffer from psoriasis may also develop psoriatic arthritis, a specific form of the disease. If left untreated, it can cause joint injury in addition to the usual symptoms of pain, stiffness, and edema. Medication, physical therapy, and changes to one's way of life are common components of treatment plans for psoriatic arthritis, with the goals of reducing inflammation and improving joint function.

Causes of Danger

Obesity, smoking, stress, specific infections (such as streptococcal infections), and a family history of the condition are some of the risk factors for getting psoriasis. Individuals can benefit from better health decision-making and risk management when aware of these risk factors.

News in the Field and Current Therapies

Investigating the causes of psoriasis and finding better ways to treat it is an active area of research.

Medications applied topically, light therapy, oral medication, biological therapies, and behavioral modifications (like management of stress and avoidance of triggers) are all part of the current treatment arsenal for psoriasis. Individuals with varying types and severity of psoriasis receive individualized treatment programs.

Managing One's Lifestyle

Lifestyle changes are just as important as medication when it comes to controlling psoriasis. Some of these measures include eating right, controlling stress, not smoking, getting plenty of exercise, avoiding environmental and drug triggers, and following a dermatologist-recommended skincare regimen. Psoriasis sufferers can lessen the frequency and severity of flare-ups and enhance their quality of life by consistently caring for themselves.

CHAPTER 2
PSORIASIS: A SCIENTIFIC PERSPECTIVE

Psoriasis and the Immune System:

In psoriasis, the immune system targets healthy skin cells as targets, leading to the development of the disease. The red, scaly patches that are characteristic of psoriasis are caused by the rapid turnover of skin cells, which is caused by an aberrant immune response. To create successful treatments for psoriasis, it is essential to understand the immune system's role in the condition.

The Role of Heredity:

Psoriasis is strongly hereditary; in fact, about 30% of those with the ailment also have a close relative who suffers from it. Some hereditary variations affect the immune system's reaction and the pace of skin cell turnover, making some people more likely to develop psoriasis. The precise genes that cause psoriasis and how they work are the subject of continuing research.

Illness and Its Function:

One of the main causes of psoriasis symptoms is inflammation. It causes redness, swelling, and itching by activating the skin's inflammatory pathways, which are caused by the immune system. To alleviate psoriasis symptoms, it is necessary to understand the function of inflammation and then create treatments that target and diminish these inflammatory responses.

The Life Cycle of Skin Cells:

Psoriasis is characterized by an abnormal skin cell growth cycle, which causes both a fast turnover and a buildup of surface skin cells. Psoriasis is characterized by the development of thick, scaly patches as a result of an accelerated growth cycle. The development of treatments that normalize skin cell growth and alleviate the severity of psoriasis symptoms can be advanced through the study of this cycle.

Immune Factor:

Psoriasis is characterized by an autoimmune reaction in which the skin's healthy cells are wrongly attacked. Understanding the efficacy of biologics and other immune system-modulating medications in psoriasis symptom management requires an appreciation of this autoimmune component.

Factors Influencing the Environment:

Environmental factors have a role in the development and worsening of psoriasis, in addition to genes and immunological dysregulation. Psoriasis symptoms can be exacerbated by factors like stress, infections, specific drugs, and lifestyle choices like smoking or high alcohol intake. Effective psoriasis management requires the identification and management of these triggers.

Conditions that occur together:

Several medical conditions, such as heart disease, metabolic syndrome, and autoimmune diseases like psoriatic arthritis, are linked to psoriasis. Care for those with psoriasis should be holistic, taking into account not only the skin symptoms but also the management of any underlying medical issues.

Social and psychological aspects:

Because of its apparent symptoms, chronic nature, and potential social stigma, psoriasis can greatly affect mental health and quality of life. People who suffer from psoriasis often struggle with mental health difficulties like low self-esteem, anxiety, depression, and stress. Psoriasis treatment that takes a holistic approach must include counseling and psychological assistance.

The Role of Hormones:

Puberty, pregnancy, and menopause are all times of hormonal change that might affect psoriasis symptoms. Hormonal fluctuations have the potential to worsen or alleviate psoriasis, demonstrating the intricate relationship between hormones and immune system activity in this disorder.

New Treatment Options:

Novel psoriasis treatments, including biologics, small compounds, and specific immune-modulating drugs, have been developed as a result of scientific advancements. Those whose psoriasis is moderate to severe and does not react well to conventional treatments may find hope in these novel remedies. People with psoriasis and their treatment outcomes and quality of life can be enhanced via ongoing research in this field.

Healthcare providers and patients afflicted by psoriasis must have a thorough understanding of the disease to effectively treat it. This includes immune system involvement, environmental triggers, and new therapeutic approaches. We can strive for better management and enhanced patient quality of life by investigating the root causes of psoriasis and taking a holistic view of the disease's effects.

CHAPTER 3

HANDLING INTENSE PSORIASIS EPISODES

The Definitive Resource for Psoriasis: Flare-Up Management

Life quality can be greatly affected by psoriasis, a skin disorder that persists over an extended period. Learning what sets off flare-ups, making positive lifestyle changes, and making use of available therapies are all part of managing the condition. A thorough overview of options for the management of psoriasis is provided in this handbook.

Things to Steer Clear of

Common Initiators

1. Stress: Exacerbations of psoriasis, or flare-ups, can be caused by psychological stress.

2. Psoriasis can be brought on or made worse by infections, such as strep throat or any number of bacteria or viruses.

3. **Skin Injuries**: New psoriasis lesions can develop after skin cuts, scrapes, or even sunburn.

4. **Dry, cold weather**: Because it dries out the skin, dry, cold weather can cause flare-ups.

5. A worsening of psoriasis symptoms has been associated with both smoking and heavy alcohol use.

6. Psoriasis can be exacerbated by some drugs, such as beta-blockers, lithium, and antimalarials.

Methods for Avoiding Danger

To lessen the likelihood of contracting an illness, it is important to practice good hygiene by regularly washing one's hands and staying away from sick people.

- **Prevent Skin Injuries**: Wear protective clothing whenever you are doing something that could hurt your skin.

Keep skin moist and use a humidifier as needed during cold, dry weather; **Monitor Weather**.

- **Reduce Alcohol Consumption and Kick the Habit of Smoking**: Get help to kick the habit of smoking and cut back on alcohol.

- **Medication Management**: Check with doctors to see if any other medications could be helpful.

Approaches to Reducing Stress

1. A great way to lower your stress levels is to practice mindfulness or meditation regularly.

2. **Practice Deep Breathing**: If you're experiencing severe stress, try these simple breathing exercises.

3. **Exercise**: The feel-good hormone endorphins are released with regular exercise, which can aid in stress reduction.

4. Cognitive Behavioural Therapy (CBT): CBT can assist in altering unhelpful ways of thinking that add to stress.

5. **Interests & Hobbies**: Taking part in things you love doing is a terrific way to relax.

6. Social support, such as spending time with loved ones or participating in a support group, can help ease emotional distress.

Nutrition and Diet Advice

A Diet that Reduces Inflammation

1. Inflammation can be alleviated by consuming fruits and vegetables, which are abundant in antioxidants.

2. Omega-3 fatty acids: Omega-3 fatty acids are anti-inflammatory and can be found in walnuts, salmon, and flaxseed.

3. **Whole Grains**: Include whole grains in your diet to aid weight maintenance and inflammation reduction.

4. Proteins that are low in fat and packed with critical nutrients can be found in lean sources like chicken, turkey, and lentils.

5. **Healthy Fats**: Consuming nuts, avocados, and olive oil can help control inflammation.

Avoiding Certain Foods

- **Processed Foods**: These foods might make inflammation worse because they are often filled with sugar and bad fats.

Because of its high saturated fat content, red meat has the potential to aggravate inflammation.

- **Dairy Products**: For some people, dairy seems to bring on their symptoms.

Inflammation and excess weight gain can be worsened by consuming foods that are high in sugar.

Alcohol: Has the potential to bring on or aggravate psoriasis flare-ups.

Daily Skincare Programme

Regular Schedule

1. **Gentle Cleaning**: To prevent irritation, use gentle, fragrance-free cleaners.

2. After a bath, lock in hydration by using a thick, fragrance-free moisturizer.

3. **Honey Routines**: To calm the skin, soak in lukewarm water with some Epsom salts, Dead Sea salts, or oils.

4. **Topical Treatments**: Follow your doctor's instructions while using any topical treatments, such as corticosteroids or vitamin D analogs.

5. **Stay Away from Harsh Products**: Things that irritate the skin include things like alcohol, perfumes, and dyes.

Sun Protection Recommendations

Advantages and Safety Measures

1. **Moderate Exposure**: As a result of UVB radiation, psoriasis symptoms can be alleviated by brief exposure to the sun.

2. To avoid sunburn, apply sunscreen even on undamaged regions. Choose an SPF 30 or greater broad-spectrum sunscreen.

3. **Time**: To lessen the likelihood of sunburn, stay out of the sun from 10 AM to 4 PM, which is peak hours.

4. To avoid sunburn, it's best to gradually increase the amount of time spent outside.

Physical fitness and regular exercise

Advantages

1. **De-Stresses**: Exercising helps alleviate tension, which is a known flare-up trigger.

2. Exercising regularly aids in weight management and cardiovascular health, which in turn improves overall health.

3. **Improves Mood**: Exercising releases feel-good endorphins, which can lift your spirits and alleviate worry and despair.

Important Hints

Walking, swimming, and yoga are low-impact activities that are easy on the skin and joints.

Stay Hydrated: To maintain hydrated skin, drink lots of water.

- **Cloth Comfortably**: To lessen skin irritation, use loose-fitting, breathable clothing.

- **Take It Easy**: To avoid hurting yourself or overworking yourself, build up to more intense and longer workouts gradually.

Sleeping Properly

Significance

1. A lack of quality sleep can worsen psoriasis and impact general health.

2. **Restorative Rest**: Getting enough sleep is important for skin health since it helps the body repair and rejuvenate.

Important Hints

- **Create a Schedule**: Every day, set an alarm for the same time and stick to it.

Keep the bedroom cool, dark, and quiet to create an environment that is conducive to relaxation.

For better sleep, **Reduce Screen Time**: Put down the phone or tablet at least an hour before bed.

If you're having trouble winding down for the night, try some relaxation techniques. Deep breathing, meditation, or even just reading a book can help.

Non-Conventional Medical Help

Alternatives

1. **Acupuncture**: By lowering stress levels and increasing blood flow, it may alleviate symptoms.

2. **Aromatherapy**: Chamomile and lavender, two essential oils, can help you unwind and feel less anxious.

3. **Herbal Supplements**: Oregon grape, turmeric, and aloe vera may alleviate inflammation and discomfort. You should always check with your doctor before beginning any new supplement regimen.

4. Some people get relief from their symptoms with **phototherapy**, which involves controlled exposure to UVB light.

The Use of OTC Drugs

Simple Solutions

1. When shopping for a moisturizer, try to find one that includes aloe vera, shea butter, or ceramides among its constituents.

2. Salicylic acid is a skin smoother and scale remover.

3. **Coal Tar**: Scalp irritation, itching, and inflammation can be alleviated with the use of coal tar, which is found in several hair care products.

4. Hydrocortisone cream is a gentle corticosteroid that helps alleviate irritation and inflammation.

Resilience Techniques

Mental and Emotional Assistance

1. Joining a support group is a great way to meet like-minded people and get some much-needed perspective.

2. The emotional toll of psoriasis can be better managed with the support of professional counseling.

3. People can have more control over their symptoms by **education**, which entails learning about the illness.

4. **Positive Self-Talk**: Remind yourself of the good things in your life and concentrate on the things you can change.

Changes to One's Way of Life

1. **Changes to Your Routine**: Make time in your day to reflect on and take care of yourself.

2. **Goal Setting**: Establish attainable, practical objectives for the management of symptoms and general well-being.

3. If you want your relationships to be healthy, you need to be around people who will encourage and understand you.

4. **Mindfulness and Acceptance**: Enhance your emotional health and resilience by cultivating these practices.

People suffering from psoriasis can greatly enhance their quality of life, control their condition, and lessen the frequency and severity of flare-ups by learning and applying these tactics.

CHAPTER 4

PSORIASIS MEDICAL TREATMENTS

Psoriasis Essentials: A Medical Professional's Guide to Treatments

A persistent autoimmune skin ailment known as psoriasis causes red, scaly patches on the skin due to the fast turnover of skin cells. How serious the problem is and how well the patient responds determine the treatment possibilities. A comprehensive guide to the several psoriasis treatments is provided below.

Aesthetic Remedies

To begin managing mild to moderate psoriasis, topical therapy is the best option. When used topically, they alleviate inflammation and delay the skin's cell turnover rate.

1. The topical drugs that are most often used for psoriasis are corticosteroids. They are effective because they dampen the immune response and decrease inflammation. There are moderate over-the-counter choices and strong prescription formulations of corticosteroids. Skin thinning and resistance are side effects that can occur with long-term use, thus they are often used in short bursts.

2. Synthetic vitamin D derivatives, such as calcipotriene (Dovonex), are useful for reducing the rate of skin cell proliferation. Combining them with corticosteroids increases their effectiveness.

3. Scalp inflammation, itching, and scaling can all be alleviated with the traditional use of coal tar. More user-friendly than earlier formulas, modern ones are also less messy and smell better.

4. **Anthralin**: This medication is used to reduce abnormalities in DNA activity in skin cells. It is effective but can irritate and discolor the skin.

5. **Topical Retinoids**: **Tazorac** and similar products are derived from vitamin A and help decrease skin cell formation and inflammation.

6. Although they are not licensed for psoriasis specifically, **calcineurin inhibitors** pimecrolimus (Elidel) and tacrolimus (Protopic) are beneficial for sensitive areas including the face and skin folds.

Photographic therapy

Under medical supervision, phototherapy—also known as light therapy—involves exposing the skin to UV light. Patients with moderate to severe psoriasis usually benefit from its usage.

1. **UVB Phototherapy**: Compared to broadband UVB, narrowband UVB is safer and more effective. For severe cases of psoriasis, it might reduce the rate of skin cell turnover.

2. **PUVA (Psoralen + UVA)**: Here, a photosensitizing medicine (psoralen) is taken before being exposed to ultraviolet A radiation. Due to the elevated risk of skin cancer, it

necessitates meticulous monitoring despite its excellent efficacy.

3. **Excimer Laser**: This phototherapy technique is ideal for localized plaques because it concentrates UVB light and applies it to specific skin locations.

Medications in the System

For moderate to severe cases of psoriasis or psoriatic arthritis, systemic therapies are administered through injections or taken orally and act systemically throughout the body.

1. The immunosuppressant methotrexate slows down the skin's cell turnover and inflammation. Because of the risk of liver damage and other adverse effects, it must be monitored regularly.

2. Closporine is an immunosuppressant that rapidly reduces the severity of psoriasis. However, it is usually prescribed for a short period only because of the risk of renal damage and high blood pressure.

3. As an oral retinoid, **Acitretin** aids in maintaining proper cell development in the skin. Though it isn't as successful as other systemic treatments, it's still a good choice for people who can't take other drugs.

Biologic medications

A biologic is a sophisticated medicinal product that originates from a live organism. These medications are used for moderate to severe cases of psoriasis and work by targeting specific areas of the immune system.

1. Medications that inhibit tumor necrosis factor-alpha, a protein that plays a role in systemic inflammation, include etanercept (Enbrel), infliximab (Remicade), and adalimumab (Humira).

2. Specific interleukins involved in psoriasis can be targeted by interleukin inhibitors. One example is secukinumab (Cosentyx), which

targets IL-17, and another is ustekinumab (Stelara), which targets IL-12 and IL-23.

Treatments in Combination

The goal of combination therapy is to increase efficacy while decreasing negative effects by utilizing two or more medicines at the same time.

1. To better manage symptoms, it can be helpful to use systemic drugs in conjunction with topical therapies such as corticosteroids or vitamin D analogs.

2. Combining phototherapy with other therapies, such as topicals or systemic medicines, can lead to more rapid and long-lasting relief.

Drugs administered intravenously

Injectable drugs include biologics and, for more serious cases, systemic therapies.

1. The main injectable therapies for psoriasis are biologics, which work by blocking particular immune mechanisms.

2. If a patient is unable to take methotrexate orally, injections are another option.

Medications Taken Orally

Psoriasis oral medicine options mostly consist of systemic anti-inflammatory and skin cell turnover regulators.

1. Oral administration of methotrexate is indicated for the treatment of severe psoriasis and psoriatic arthritis.

2. Because of its strong immunosuppressive effects, **Cyclosporine** is only used for short-term treatments.

3. **Acitretin**: A retinoid that can be taken orally and is appropriate for long-term use in specific individuals.

Anti-inflammatory drugs

One way to treat inflammation is using corticosteroids, which can be injected, taken orally, or applied topically.

1. For localized psoriasis, **Topical Corticosteroids** can alleviate inflammation and irritation.

2. **Systemic Corticosteroids**: Psoriasis patients should typically avoid injectable or oral formulations of these drugs because of the risk of severe rebound flares.

** Immunomodulators**

You can get immunomodulators in both topical and systemic forms, and they work by adjusting the immune response.

1. For sensitive skin, try tacrolimus or pimecrolimus, two topical calcineurin inhibitors.

2. Important systemic options include methotrexate and cyclosporine, which are immunomodulators.

Guidelines for Treatment

Guidelines for the treatment of psoriasis include a progressive strategy that takes into account the severity of the disease and the patient's reaction.

1. The initial line of defense against mild psoriasis is topical therapies; in severe cases, phototherapy may be used.

2. Systemic meds and biologics, ideally used in combination, are advised for moderate to severe psoriasis.

3. **Patient-Centered Approach**: By taking into account aspects such as comorbidities, lifestyle, and treatment preferences, treatments should be customized to meet the unique needs of each patient.

4. Systemic and biological treatments, in particular, necessitate constant vigilance for adverse effects and treatment effectiveness.

Finally, a personalized and all-encompassing strategy combining topical, phototherapy, systemic, and biologic therapies is necessary for the management of psoriasis. To get the best possible results and enhance the quality of life, patients and healthcare providers must work closely together.

CHAPTER 5

COMPREHENSIVE METHODS FOR TREATING PSORIASIS

Meditation and Mindfulness

An Introduction to Meditation and Mindfulness:

Becoming fully present in the here and now, without attaching any judgment to it, is the practice of mindfulness. Meditation is an integral part of mindfulness since it is a set of practices that can help you focus your attention and relax your mind.

Psoriasis Benefits:

Psoriasis symptoms might be brought on or worsened by stress, according to research. Psoriasis flare-ups may be less severe and less frequent if you practice mindfulness and meditation, which lower stress levels. People with long-term illnesses, such as psoriasis, can benefit from their increased emotional health, decreased anxiety, and better quality of life.

Finding method:

- **Mindful Breathing:** Bringing awareness to the breath as a means of grounding oneself in the here and now.

- **Body Scan Meditation:** Concentrating on the felt sensations in your entire body, from your head to your toes.

- **Guided Imagery:** Creating mental pictures to ease tension and divert attention away from unpleasant sensations.

Putting into Practice in Everyday Life:

Take it easy for a few minutes each day at first, and work your way up to longer sessions. Guided sessions can be found in apps and online resources, which are great for beginners.

Acupressure and Acupuncture

How Acupressure and Acupuncture Work:

To promote healing, acupuncture practitioners inject very thin needles into certain anatomical locations. Acupressure is based on the same principles as acupuncture but employs finger pressure rather than needles.

Psoriasis Benefits:

The traditional belief is that these methods can help alleviate tension, increase blood flow, and return the body's energy balance (Qi). They have the potential to reduce inflammation, discomfort, and itching caused by psoriasis.

Typical sessions:

- **Acupuncture:** After a trained professional inserts needles into certain sites, the patient is typically allowed some time to relax.

- **Acupressure:** This therapeutic modality entails the application of pressure to specific anatomical sites, either by a trained professional or by the patient.

Factors to Think About:

To avoid hazards like infections or poor technique, be sure treatments are delivered by certified professionals.

Natural Treatments

Analysing Natural Treatments:

The use of compounds derived from plants for therapeutic purposes is known as herbal medicines. Analgesic and anti-inflammatory effects are found in numerous plants.

Common Herbs Used to Treat Psoriasis:

The calming and hydrating properties of aloe vera make it a popular skincare ingredient.

Turmeric: The anti-inflammatory effects of curcumin are found in turmeric.

Helps decrease inflammation and slow down the proliferation of skin cells; **Mahonia Aquifolium (Oregon Grape)** is one such plant.

Tea Tree Oil: It can alleviate skin irritation thanks to its anti-inflammatory and antibacterial characteristics.

How to Use It and How Much to Take:

You can consume herbal supplements or use them topically for relief. To make sure you are getting the right dosage and are not putting yourself at risk, talk to your doctor before beginning any herbal medication.

Numerous Ayurvedic Methods

Getting to Know Ayurveda:

Diet, lifestyle, and natural remedies are the cornerstones of Ayurveda, an old Indian medical system that seeks to balance the body's energy (doshas).

Psoriasis Treatment from an Ayurvedic Perspective:

- **Eating Plan:** Prioritises low-IgG foods while cutting down inflammatory culprits like processed, spicy, and acidic foods.

- Purgation, massage, and herbal steam baths are all part of the detoxification process, which is also known as panchakarma.

- **Natural Remedies:** Harnessing the anti-inflammatory and cleansing powers of herbs such as guggul, neem, and turmeric.

Advice on the Way of Life:

To promote health and harmony among the doshas, it is essential to practice yoga, meditate regularly, and stick to a regular sleep pattern.

fragrance treatment
Aromatherapy Concepts:

Aromatherapy is a form of alternative medicine that promotes mental and physical health through the use of therapeutic essential oils derived from plants.

Psoriasis Benefits:**

A person's emotional and skin health can both benefit from the use of essential oils, which have anti-inflammatory, anti-stress, and itching properties.

Aromatherapy Essential Oils:

The sedative and anti-inflammatory properties of lavender have made it a popular choice.

Chamomile: Assists in soothing irritated skin and fostering a sense of calm.

The anti-inflammatory and antibacterial effects of eucalyptus are well-documented.

Methods for Application:

Use essential oils topically, in a bath, or diffused into the air after diluting with a carrier oil. Make sure there are no adverse responses by doing a patch test.

Treatments using Homoeopathy

The Basics of Homoeopathy:

Holistically, homeopathy employs extremely dilute chemicals to arouse the body's recuperative mechanisms.

Homeopathic Treatments for Psoriasis:

If you have dry, scaly skin, try the Arsenicum album.

- Graphites are used for skins that are thick and ooze.

If you're experiencing itching or burning, try using sulfur.

Analysis and Administration:

Homeopathic medicines are individualized based on each patient's symptoms and health status, therefore it's best to see a trained homeopath for a unique treatment plan.

Doing Tai Chi and Yoga

Getting to Know Tai Chi and Yoga:

Both are old ways of healing that include physical postures, breathing exercises, and meditation.

Psoriasis Benefits:

Psoriasis symptoms can be better managed with regular practice, which reduces stress, improves immunological function, and enhances physical fitness.

Practices that are suggested:

*Yoga**: **Yin** and **Hatha** are two gentle forms of yoga that emphasize stretching and relaxation.

Tai Chi entails meditation, slow, deliberate movement, and deep breathing.

Working into Everyday Routines:

Begin with more basic activities and work your way up to more complex ones by taking introductory classes or using online instructions. Strive for consistent, regular practice.

Massage Treatments

A Guide to Massage Therapy:

For relaxation, pain relief, and stress reduction, massage entails applying pressure to specific areas of the body's soft tissues.

Psoriasis Benefits:

Massage has many health benefits, including better circulation, less stress, and healthier skin through increased toxin clearance and better immune function.

Massages and Their Kinds:

- **Swedish Massage:** A soothing method that can help alleviate tension and anxiety.

Deep Tissue Massage: This type of massage targets the deepest layers of muscle, which can help alleviate persistent discomfort.

Aromatherapy Massage: Enhances the therapeutic benefits of massage by incorporating essential oils.

Factors to Think About:

If you let your therapist know that you suffer from psoriasis, they can modify their methods to be gentler on your skin.

Natural Health Care

Discovering the Field of Naturopathic Medicine:

Holistic treatment is the hallmark of naturopathy, which emphasizes natural cures and the body's healing abilities.

Methods for Dealing with Psoriasis:

- **Nutrition and Diet:** Tailored eating regimens to alleviate inflammation and promote radiant skin.

To help the immune system work better and alleviate symptoms, you can take **supplements** including vitamins, minerals, and herbs.

- **Changes in Lifestyle:** Managing stress, exercising regularly, and getting enough sleep to improve health in general.

Application Review:

Collaborate with a qualified naturopathic physician to design a thorough and tailored treatment regimen.

Integrative health care

A Comprehensive Overview of Integrative Medicine:

To address the full patient, integrative medicine integrates traditional medicine with complementary therapies supported by scientific evidence.

Methods for Dealing with Psoriasis:

Traditional Methods of Treatment: Medications are given systemically, phototherapy, and topical applications.

Complementary Therapies: Alterations to one's food, acupuncture, herbal treatments, and practices of mindfulness to improve one's health as a whole and alleviate symptoms.

What are the advantages?

It provides a more tailored and efficient treatment plan by taking a holistic approach that considers both the patient's physical and mental health.

CHAPTER 6

EMOTIONAL WELL-BEING AND PSORIASIS

Psoriasis's Effect on Mental Health

The emotional toll of psoriasis is just as substantial as the physical ones. Embarrassment, humiliation, or self-consciousness may set in due to its chronic nature and the fact that it is visible. Your relationships, productivity at work, and general happiness can all take a hit when you're feeling down.

Dealing with Difficult Emotions

It is essential to establish coping mechanisms to handle emotional difficulties. Mindfulness, writing in a journal, and pursuing interests might help you feel more in control and divert your attention from unpleasant thoughts.

Counselling and Support Groups

By bringing people together in support groups, those going through tough times might find understanding and compassion from those who have been there themselves. Helping people overcome emotional obstacles and learn new coping mechanisms is one of the many wonderful goals of counseling, whether it's individual or group sessions.

Methods for Reducing Stress

Effective therapy of psoriasis requires attention to stress. Psoriasis sufferers may get relief from their symptoms if they practice stress reduction techniques such as deep breathing, yoga, meditation, or regular exercise.

Developing Confidence

Acknowledging and valuing one's qualities and achievements is an important step in developing self-esteem. A healthier self-image is the result of regular self-care, goal-setting, and positive self-talk.

De-escalating Depression and Anxiety

Psoriasis sufferers sometimes struggle with mental health issues like anxiety and sadness. It is crucial to get treatment from a professional, whether it's therapy or medication when needed. Another factor that can have a favorable effect on mental health is making adjustments to one's lifestyle, such as eating better and exercising more frequently.

Mental-Physical Link

The importance of one's emotional and mental well-being on one's physical health is highlighted by the mind-body connection. Mindfulness meditation, relaxation methods, and cognitive-behavioral therapy are some practices that can alleviate psoriasis symptoms while also improving mental health.

Activities for Healing

Art therapy, music therapy, or just being outside in nature can have a calming and restorative effect. Participating in these pursuits can help one unwind, express themselves, and learn more about themselves.

Setting Objectives and Maintaining an Upbeat Attitude

A person's resilience and drive can be enhanced by setting attainable goals and keeping an optimistic attitude. A more positive outlook can be developed via the practice of thankfulness and the celebration of minor successes.

Considering Expert Advice

Last but not least, if you want your psoriasis under control, you need to contact a doctor. Individualized treatment programs, encompassing medicine, counseling, and lifestyle suggestions, can be provided by psychologists, dermatologists, and other medical professionals.

One way to help people with psoriasis manage their illness and improve their overall health is to treat the psychological components of it with empathy, understanding, and comprehensive care.

CHAPTER 7
UNIQUE GROUPS AFFECTED BY PSORIASIS

Exploring Psoriasis During Pregnancy

Finding an effective therapy for psoriasis while pregnant can be challenging because of the necessity to ensure the fetus's well-being. It is commonly believed that hormonal changes during pregnancy alleviate psoriasis symptoms for many people. However, psoriasis can flare up or even develop during pregnancy in rare instances. The possible effects of treatment alternatives on the pregnancy must be carefully considered. It is essential to be closely monitored by healthcare specialists during pregnancy, and topical therapies, such as corticosteroids, are often favored over systemic drugs.

Treatment for Psoriasis in Children

Due to their growing bodies and distinct psychological requirements, children with psoriasis necessitate specialized treatment. Considerations such as the child's age, symptom intensity, and quality of life impact should inform treatment choices. Mild treatments, like emollients and topical corticosteroids with low strength, are prioritized. Under strict medical supervision, systemic therapies are typically administered to patients with very severe instances. Because psoriasis can impact a child's sense of self-worth and social connections, they must receive psychological support.

Psoriasis in the Elderly

Skin changes associated with aging, co-morbidities, and drug interactions all contribute to unique difficulties in treating psoriasis in the elderly. Aiming for symptom control and increased quality of life, treatment regimens should consider these elements. Because of the risk of adverse effects and drug interactions, systemic treatments should be approached with caution, in contrast to topical therapy. To make necessary adjustments to treatment and address any new concerns quickly, healthcare providers must evaluate patients regularly.

Disparities between the Sexes and Psoriasis

Disparities between the sexes in psoriasis manifest in different ways, react differently to treatment, and have different effects on patients' quality of life. When it comes to psoriasis, men are more likely to develop it at a younger age and may have more severe symptoms, particularly on their chest and scalp. Contrarily, psoriasis severity might vary among women because of hormonal changes during menopause, pregnancy, and other similar periods. Treatment plans and support techniques can be more successfully tailored when these variances are understood.

Psoriasis Among Diverse Ethnic Communities

The intensity, distribution, and response to therapies for psoriasis might vary across ethnic groups. Hyperpigmentation or post-inflammatory changes, for example, may be more apparent in people of darker skin tone than redness. Treatment adherence and the perceived stigma of visible skin disorders are influenced by cultural factors as well. Optimal treatment can only be delivered by healthcare professionals who are attuned to these subtleties.

Psoriasis and the LGBTQ+ Community

Social stigma, mental health issues, and healthcare access are disproportionately burdensome for LGBTQ+ members living with psoriasis. It is crucial to implement inclusive and affirmative care practices so that people with psoriasis can feel comfortable talking about their condition and their treatment options in a safe setting. Improving treatment outcomes and general well-being can be achieved by customizing treatment regimens to meet varied identities and lifestyles.

Treatment of Psoriasis in Long-Term Conditions

Psoriatic arthritis, diabetes, and cardiovascular disease are among the chronic illnesses that frequently occur alongside psoriasis. A team of experts, including dermatologists and rheumatologists, is needed to manage psoriasis when it is associated with these other conditions. It is important to think about how psoriasis therapies might affect other health issues when developing a treatment plan, and the same goes for other health issues. For the best possible management, healthcare providers must work closely together and monitor patients often.

Psoriasis and Being Overweight

It is well-known that obesity and psoriasis are related, and that the two diseases affect each other's development and severity. The metabolic alterations and systemic inflammation caused by obesity can make psoriasis worse. Insulin resistance and excess weight may be associated with inflammation in psoriasis. Managing weight and making dietary adjustments are examples of lifestyle alterations that can enhance health outcomes and work in tandem with psoriasis therapies.

Psoriasis's Effects on Sexual Health

Sexual health, intimacy, and self-confidence are all negatively impacted by psoriasis. Sexual dysfunction and relationship issues can be exacerbated by genital involvement, psychological anxiety, and visible psoriatic plaques. Addressing physical discomfort, emotional well-being, and treatment preferences requires an open conversation about sexual difficulties with healthcare practitioners. Help from counseling and support groups could be useful for people dealing with these challenges.

Things to Think About at Work

When dealing with psoriasis at work, it's important to think about making adjustments, being transparent, and managing apparent symptoms. Psoriasis education for employers and coworkers can help create a more accepting workplace. Having the ability to work remotely or have their schedules changed can greatly assist individuals in managing their treatment schedules and reducing stress levels. To further improve workplace wellness, it is important to underline the significance of self-care and methods for managing stress.

All of these points show how unique psoriasis care is for different groups of people, and how important it is to provide each patient with individualized, comprehensive care. To improve the quality of life and optimize results for individuals with psoriasis, healthcare practitioners, patients, and support networks must collaborate.

CHAPTER 8
WAYS TO MANAGE PSORIASIS IN YOUR DAILY LIFE

The Definitive Resource for Living Well with Psoriasis

Nutrition & Diet in the Treatment of Psoriasis

When dealing with psoriasis, it's important to have a balanced diet. To lessen the frequency and severity of flare-ups, try eating more anti-inflammatory foods such as fresh produce, whole grains, lean meats, and fruits. Fish, flaxseeds, and walnuts are good sources of omega-3 fatty acids. Red meat, processed foods, and sugary snacks are trigger foods that you should try to avoid if you want your symptoms to go away even more.

Quitting Smoking and Alcohol

Psoriasis symptoms might be worsened by smoking and alcohol. Improving skin health can be as simple as cutting less on alcohol and smoking. People might get help in the form of counseling and support groups as they work to quit.

Tips for Taking Care of Your Skin

To control psoriasis, it is necessary to use gentle skincare products. Moisturizers and gentle cleansers that do not contain fragrances are ideal for maintaining skin moisture. Hot water and harsh soaps might aggravate symptoms, so it's best to avoid them. Sunscreens with high SPF values are also effective in shielding the skin from harmful UV radiation.

Options for Attire

To alleviate the itching and discomfort that psoriasis can cause, it's best to dress in loose, airy garments. Choose loose-fitting garments that won't irritate the skin and go for cotton or other soft fibres instead. Keep in mind that certain garments may irritate delicate skin due to their tags and seams.

Changes to the Environment

Improving the quality of life for those living with psoriasis can be achieved by making home adjustments. To avoid skin dryness, keep the temperature and humidity moderate. When the weather gets dry, use a humidifier to keep your skin from drying out, and stay away from products with harsh ingredients.

Overcoming Psoriasis on the Road

Preparation is key while traveling with psoriasis. Be sure to bring your medications, necessary skincare products, and plenty of comfortable clothing. Before you go, find out where the nearest medical facilities are in case you have any problems or emergencies. To get assistance, let your traveling partners know about your problem.

Caring for Your Money

The expense of skincare products, doctor appointments, and medication to manage psoriasis can add up. Look into medication assistance programs and insurance to see if you might get some financial relief. Healthcare spending can be better managed with a budget and some planning.

Emotional Well-being and Eczema

For mental health, it's crucial to keep in touch with friends and family. If you want your loved ones to be more sympathetic and supportive, educate them about psoriasis. Find ways to improve your sense of self-worth and confidence, such as taking up a new hobby or becoming a member of a support group.

Relationship Management

Maintaining healthy relationships while managing psoriasis requires honest and open communication To foster empathy and understanding, talk to those you care about about how you're feeling. Partner involvement in treatment planning and mutual support in times of need should be encouraged.

Thoughts on What May Come Next

Keeping track of psoriasis symptoms and how well treatment is working is an important part of long-term planning. Build a thorough care plan in conjunction with your healthcare providers. For the best care of psoriasis, stay up-to-date on new treatment options and research advances.

CHAPTER 9

HEALTHCARE SYSTEM NAVIGATION

Choosing a Reliable Medical Professional

To effectively manage psoriasis, it is essential to find the correct healthcare professional. Look into rheumatologists or dermatologists who have treated psoriasis before. Find a specialist who is well-respected by their patients and has board certification. Their accessibility, availability, communication style, and practice location are all important considerations.

Successfully Interacting with Medical Professionals

To get the most out of your treatment, it's important to talk to your doctor. Take notes on your symptoms, concerns, and questions before your appointments to ensure you are well-prepared. Give a detailed account of your symptoms, noting their intensity and any things that seem to bring them on. Inquire about the whole range of treatment options, including any risks and how they will be managed in the long run.

Expert Opinions and Second Opinions

Do not hesitate to consult with another competent expert for a second opinion if you have any doubts regarding your diagnosis or proposed course of therapy. They might have some fresh perspectives or ideas that could be useful. Expertise in the treatment of psoriasis can be best provided by dermatologists, rheumatologists, and immunologists, among others.

Insurance Coverage Made Clear

To avoid financial hardship when obtaining psoriasis treatments, it is crucial to understand your insurance coverage. Find out what kinds of medical care, such as prescriptions, office visits, and procedures, are covered by reviewing your coverage. To get more information about your coverage and any possible out-of-pocket expenses, you might want to talk to an insurance agent or a financial counselor.

Getting Drugs and Treatments

You need to coordinate with your healthcare practitioner, pharmacist, and insurance company to access psoriasis drugs and treatments. Collaborate closely with your physician to ascertain the optimal pharmaceutical regimen, which may involve phototherapy, systemic drugs, biologic medicines, or topical treatments. Always read the label, look out for possible side effects, and know what to look out for when taking medication.

Patient Rights and Advocacy

You have the power to speak out for yourself and your healthcare requirements as a psoriasis patient. Learn about the patient's rights to privacy, confidentiality, and informed consent as they pertain to their medical records. Reach out to patient advocacy groups or legal aid agencies for assistance if you face prejudice or other forms of discrimination.

Online Medical Care and Health Technology

Psoriasis consultations, follow-ups, and monitoring are now more convenient than ever before thanks to telemedicine and digital health platforms. Look into dermatology-specific telemedicine platforms or your healthcare provider's telemedicine offerings. For virtual visits, make sure you have the right equipment, including a stable internet connection and a gadget that can handle them.

Clinical Trials and Involvement in Research

You can help find a better therapy and learn more about psoriasis by taking part in research and clinical trials. Find out whether any clinical trials could help your condition by talking to your doctor. Before you decide to participate in a study, be sure you understand all of the potential outcomes, advantages, and ethical concerns.

Medical Facilities and Urgent Care

Seek immediate medical assistance at a hospital or emergency room in the event of a severe flare-up or complications associated with psoriasis. Get to know the local healthcare facilities and hospitals that can treat psoriasis crises. Make sure to have all of your important medical records on hand in case of an emergency. This includes your diagnosis, prescriptions, and any allergies you may have.

Planning for the End of Life

Although psoriasis mostly manifests as joint and skin inflammation, it is crucial to think about end-of-life preparation as part of holistic healthcare treatment. Have a conversation with your loved ones and doctors about your wishes for end-of-life care. Make your wishes known when it matters most about your healthcare by drafting an advance directive, such as a living will or a healthcare proxy.

Proactively communicating, making educated decisions, and advocating for the best care and support are essential when navigating the healthcare system for psoriasis. Effective psoriasis management requires patient engagement, teamwork with healthcare providers, and making the most of available resources.

CHAPTER 10
TAKING CONTROL OF YOUR PSORIASIS

Resources for Learning and Research

It is through education that psoriasis can be better understood. You may find a wealth of information regarding psoriasis—its causes, symptoms, triggers, treatment options, and management strategies—in a variety of trustworthy resources. All of these resources—online platforms, medical literature, support groups, and healthcare providers—can be quite helpful to patients.

Taking Responsibility for Your Health

One way to take responsibility for one's health is to be an active participant in one's therapy. Maintaining frequent meetings with healthcare providers, taking medications as prescribed, living a healthy lifestyle, and dealing with stress are all part of this. Psoriasis can be better managed and general health can be enhanced by persons taking proactive measures.

Setting Achievable Objectives

The key to successful psoriasis management is setting attainable goals. A better quality of life, less frequent flare-ups, more mobility, or smoother skin could be among these objectives. Individuals can maintain motivation and concentrate on their path to improved health by establishing attainable objectives.

Developing a System of Mutual Assistance

When dealing with psoriasis, it helps to have people you can lean on in times of need. People in this network could include loved ones, acquaintances, medical professionals, support groups, and communities online. A sense of community, sound guidance, and emotional support can all come from talking to people who have been through similar things.

Raising Awareness about Psoriasis

Psoriasis advocates are vital in getting the word out about the condition and getting people to accept and understand it. Anyone can be an advocate by speaking out about their experiences, joining awareness campaigns, donating to research projects, and demanding better healthcare access.

The Importance of Prioritising Your Health

Psoriasis management and general health benefit greatly from self-care practices. A good diet, frequent exercise, stress reduction strategies, adequate sleep, and avoiding things that bring on symptoms are all part of this. Self-care gives people the tools they need to manage their health and make positive changes in their lives.

"Rejoicing in Success"

To keep a happy attitude and stay motivated, it is necessary to celebrate accomplishments, no matter how minor. Acknowledging and appreciating successes, whether they be treatment milestones, improved stress management, or personal objectives, can increase resilience and self-confidence.

Sustaining Oneself and Being Flexible

Being resilient and adaptable is essential for living with psoriasis. It may be necessary to attempt new treatments, make changes to one's lifestyle, reach out for help when required, and keep a positive attitude to cope with the condition's physical and emotional difficulties. Living with psoriasis isn't always smooth sailing, but building resilience and adaptation can help.

Discovering Happiness and Success

It is possible to have a happy and fulfilling life despite having psoriasis. Pursuing interests and hobbies, spending time with loved ones, being grateful, doing meaningful work, and concentrating on what makes you happy and fulfilled are all ways to achieve this.

Managing Psoriasis in a Healthy Way

Finding a happy medium is key to managing psoriasis properly. A healthy lifestyle, good symptom management, attention to emotional health, support systems, knowledge of treatment alternatives, and self-care practices are all part of this. Psoriasis does not have to define a person's life if they take the correct approach.

www.ingramcontent.com/pod-product-compliance
Lightning Source LLC
Chambersburg PA
CBHW071837210526
45479CB00001B/177